Natural Cures for Constipation

Curing Constipation Permanently

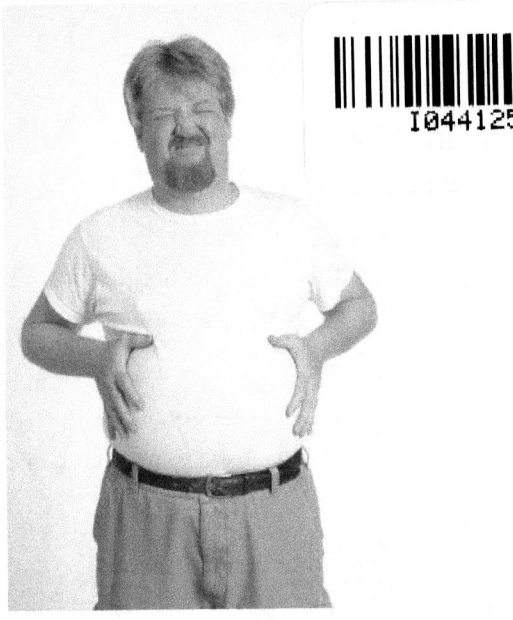

I0441250

Healthy Learning series

Dueep Jyot Singh

Mendon Cottage Books

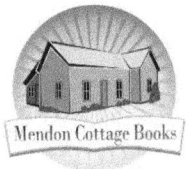

JD-Biz Publishing

All Rights Reserved.

Disclaimer

The information is this book is provided for informational purposes only. It is not intended to be used and medical advice or a substitute for proper medical treatment by a qualified health care provider. The information is believed to be accurate as presented based on research by the author.

The contents have not been evaluated by the U.S. Food and Drug Administration or any other Government or Health Organization and the contents in this book are not to be used to treat cure or prevent disease.

The author or publisher is not responsible for the use or safety of any diet, procedure or treatment mentioned in this book. The author or publisher is not responsible for errors or omissions that may exist.

Warning

The Book is for informational purposes only and before taking on any diet, treatment or medical procedure, it is recommended to consult with your primary health care provider.

Our books are available at

1. Amazon.com

2. Barnes and Noble

3. Itunes

4. Kobo

5. Smashwords

6. Google Play Books

Table of Contents

Introduction..4

How Does Constipation Happen..5

Symptoms of Constipation...7

Reasons for Chronic Constipation 10

Increasing your liquid intake..13

Water Therapy...15

Irregular Bowel Movement Habits...17

Sedentary Lifestyles...20

Factors Encouraging Constipation 24

Curing Constipation Naturally 27

Diet..29

Ripe Guavas 30

Carrots and Citrus Fruits 34

Gooseberries...36

Apples 38

Conclusion 39

Author Bio...41

Publisher..52

Introduction

Constipation is one of the ailments besetting mankind down the ages. Believe it or not, there were ancient Eastern medical treatises written in olden days, which had about 236 natural remedies to cure constipation. So for a person who is lucky enough not to know what constipation is, it is not being able to empty the elementary canal naturally and regularly. This is a condition usually accompanied with hard fecal nodules.

Constipation is one of the elements, which is often a part of human discussion, especially in social gatherings. When people begin to talk about their health, the conversation is going to go around to anybody asking the audience if they know any cure for constipation. Well brought up people may think this rather vulgar, but that is how matters stand. Nevertheless, as every human being has faced this problem sometime or the other in his life, it is an integral part of the social and natural identity of mankind.

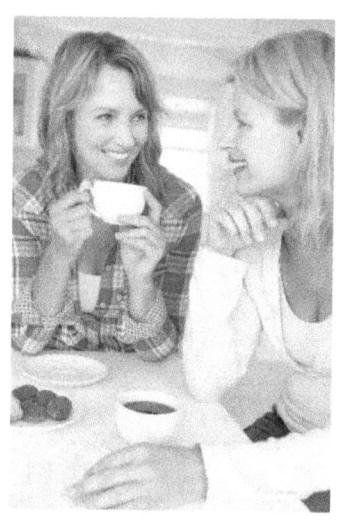

How Does Constipation Happen

The ancients always believed in having their meals at a regular time. This would make their body accustomed to digesting the food intake in a systematic manner at the proper time. That is why if people began eating their meals at different times, the whole system would have gone awry. This would prevent the waste from accumulating in the bowels at the proper time and being eliminated in a regular fashion.

In other words, if you had your meals at breakfast at 9 o'clock, lunch at 1 o'clock, Tea at 4 o'clock, dinner at 8 o'clock, your system would know all about the time when you would ingest food. It could then set up its own process of digesting the food within a given time limit, and by next morning you would have enough of that food waste ready to eliminate.

However, if you skipped breakfast, lunch to 12 o'clock, had a snack at 1 o'clock, had something else at 5 o'clock, had a large dinner at 9 o'clock and then had an after dinner snack before going to bed, your whole system would be put out of tune. Your stomach which should have been busy digesting the food you ingested would immediately be subjected to another inflow of something else which it had to digest. Within 3 days, you would be suffering from constipation.

This means that your stomach would have got rid of some waste, but they would still be something left behind in the alimentary canal and in the intestines. That was the half digested food. That means this food which was full of toxic wastes, would continue sitting in the alimentary canal, until it had to be eliminated due to the pressure of more half digested food, nodules making their appearance as you kept eating.

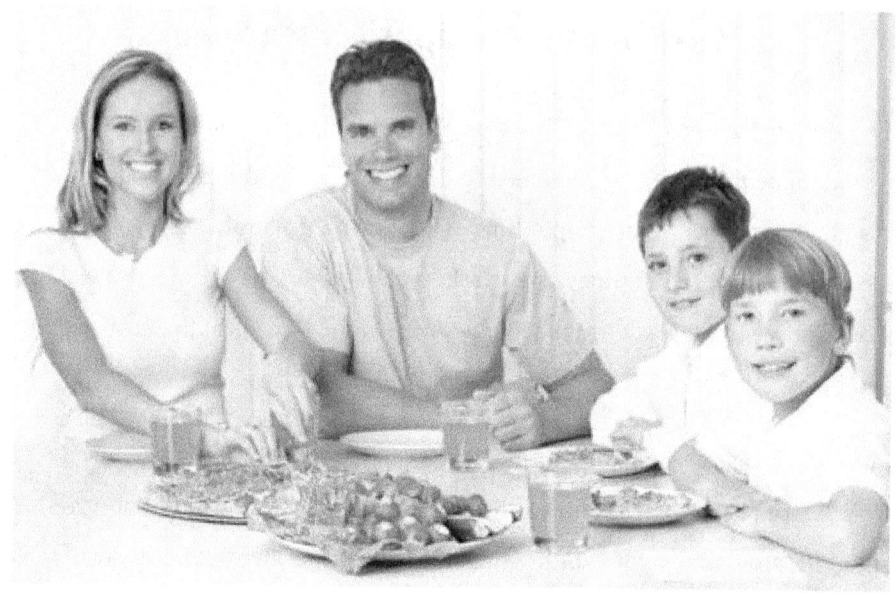

Regular healthy meals, at regular times, means good health throughout your life.

People in many parts of the world have this habit of fasting, either for health reasons or for religious reasons. They think that this is a good way to prevent constipation because no waste matter is being produced in the stomach because after all, they are not eating anything. However, when they take an enema, the bowels are emptied out with a lot of waste, which had been present in the alimentary canal. This may have been the main reason for their constipation.

Symptoms of Constipation

Imagine all that waste collecting in your stomach over a long period of time. It is not being eliminated, because there is not enough of waste present, which can be expelled from the body naturally. That is why people suffering from malnutrition are also going to be constipated, because they do not eat enough of food for the bowels to work properly.

Total starvation is going to cause the shrinking of the intestines, because they have not been given enough of food for a long while. That is why people will have been suffering from malnutrition and starvation for a long period of time are given only tiny meals often so that the stomach and get used to the process of digestion and elimination yet once again.

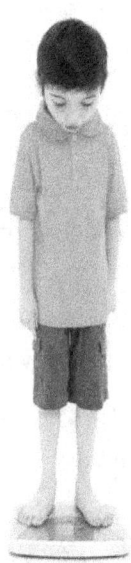

Parents being careless about the children's diets may cause the children to suffer from malnutrition and nutrient deficiency.

If a person is suffering from constipation, the food which has accumulated in his digestive system is going to start "rotting" in the normal temperature of the stomach, and the presence of moisture. This is going to form gases.

The toxins which are present in the same rotting food are going to weaken the whole system. That is because they have contaminated the blood and that blood is going to circulate throughout the whole body effectively "poisoning" it. This is going to make the body vulnerable to diseases. It is also going to make it susceptible to constipation related problems like dyspepsia, bloating, nausea, lethargy, and other problems. You may also feel yourself feeling tired, fatigued, and dull.

People suffering from constipation are definitely not chirpy and eager beavers. Their main aim in life is to get their system working properly and that is going to be the whole top priority activity in their lives. If you find yourself suffering from excess of saliva, especially when speaking, it is possible that your system is not working properly.

That is why, when we were children, and our elders found us spitting when we talked or if they found us suffering from halitosis, we were immediately given huge doses of fresh lemon juice, lots of fruit, and vegetables in order to get our stomachs working properly.

You may also find yourself feeling a bit feverish, when you are suffering from constipation. This is going to happen because there is plenty of poisonous material in your stomach busy making toxins 24/7 which have to be gotten rid of as soon as possible. And that is why you find yourself using all sorts of measures to get rid of that waste in your stomach.

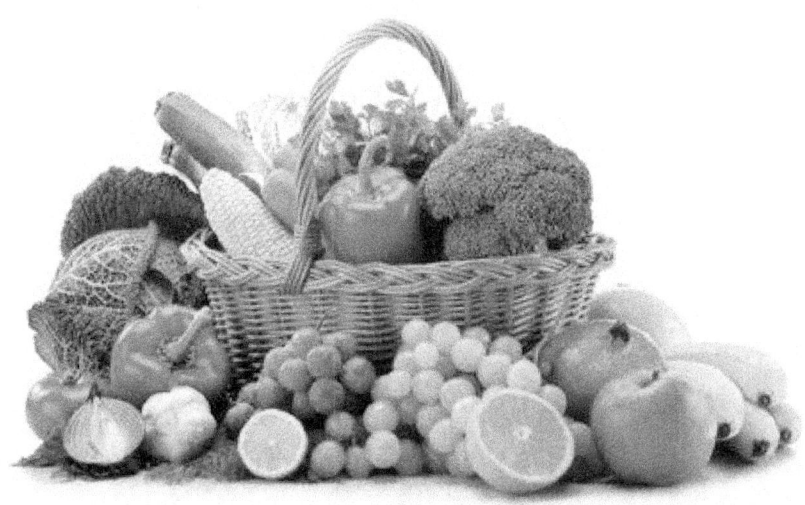

Remember that chronic constipation can give rise to piles and sciatica.

Reasons for Chronic Constipation

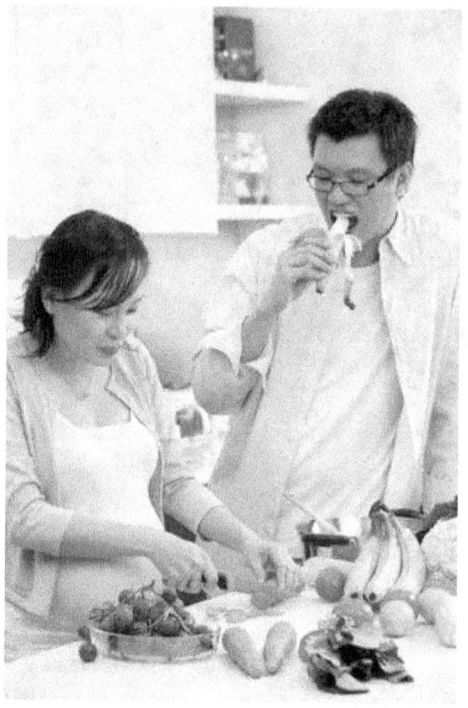

Healthy eating habits in parents mean healthier future generations.

Here are some reasons for chronic constipation, which a number of you are going to understand and sympathize with, because after all, you have gone through the same experience at least once in your lives.

I remember suffering from constipation always during the holiday season. That is because I am invited to so many social gatherings where I have to eat and drink. Even if I take little amounts of food, this unusual food intake which is quite different from my normal diet is going to upset the whole system. This food is rich, spicy, and delicious, and that is going to tempt me to eat even more than my regular normal diet. Also, I am going to eat more than usual, because that food is so absolutely mouthwatering. What happens then? One month of the holiday season, and I have to get back to my normal diet. But I have found that when I take my regular meals, I am feeling hungry. Why is it so? That is because I have been accustomed to stuffing myself during the past month on huge meals. My stomach has gotten accustomed to that amount of food, and is considering my normal diet to be possibly a starvation diet. The more you eat, the more you feel hungry. This is a normal natural state.

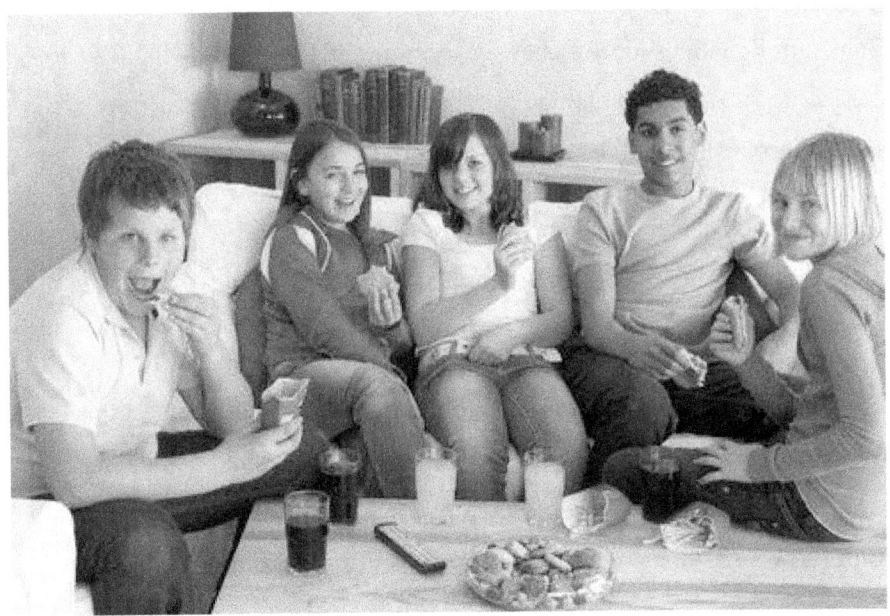

Also, we do not bother too much about what we are eating, especially when we are in company. Junk food and fast food is the norm of the day.

I have been loading myself on party food, – most of it junk – because after all, my host is paying for it, but my stomach is going to pay for it in the end! We do not bother much about diet or the composition of the food items we gobble, because they are right there in front of us, and we are not going to let that last shrimp eggroll fall to someone else's share.

And we do not bother much about spice, the richness of the food, and whether it has been made of refined flour or not. After that, we are going to down plenty of cold drinks. Also, we are in such a hurry to finish up everything in our plate, before going in for seconds – and incidentally grabbing hose vol au vents before anybody else pounces on hem – that we forget to chew. It is "take a huge bite, chew once, twice, thrice, and then gulp down." We definitely do not have the time or the inclination to follow Benjamin Franklin's idea of chewing 30 times, before swallowing. We are not inclined to act like chipmunks at parties, chewing away, when we are in such a hurry to grab all the nuts, no pun or double entendre intended.

Now this food has definitely not been mixed up with saliva in order to make it more easy to digest. In fact, the food morsels which have just reached the stomach are not broken down properly and finely.

The stomach is going to have a little bit of problem trying to digest this, because the salivary enzymes which should have been mixed in the food, along with the saliva are not present there. So the stomach has to make do with its own enzymes like pepsin, trypsin, and amylase.

Increasing your liquid intake

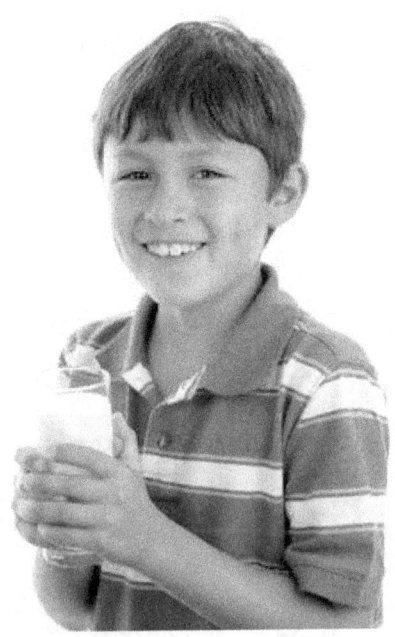

So you started on your journey to constipation by bolting down the food without chewing it. You also took it in large dollops in harried and hurried mouthfuls and in large quantities. You also kept swallowing air while bolting this food, and this air is also going to cause dyspepsia and gas in your stomach.

This is not my own imagination or invention. The ancients knew it! And they talked about it. According to them, one ate food at leisure chewing like a contented bovine, and swallowing the food without any water to aid in the digesting process. Water was always drunk half an hour before meals or in sips during the meal, to give the stomach enough of watery content in which the food could be mixed in a paste called chyme.

This chyme would be a semifluidic mass, a mixture of gastric juices, water, the food content and it would be digested partially in the stomach. After that, it would pass into the intestines, including the duodenum and the ileum . All the liquid content would be absorbed by these organs until a solid mass reached the bowels which would then be eliminated as waste.

So remember, the more liquids you take during the day, the less chance you have of getting constipated. I would suggest fresh juice, because not only is it healthy, but also, you are not poisoning your system with cocaine leaf and caffeine laced soft carbonated drinks, tea, or coffee.

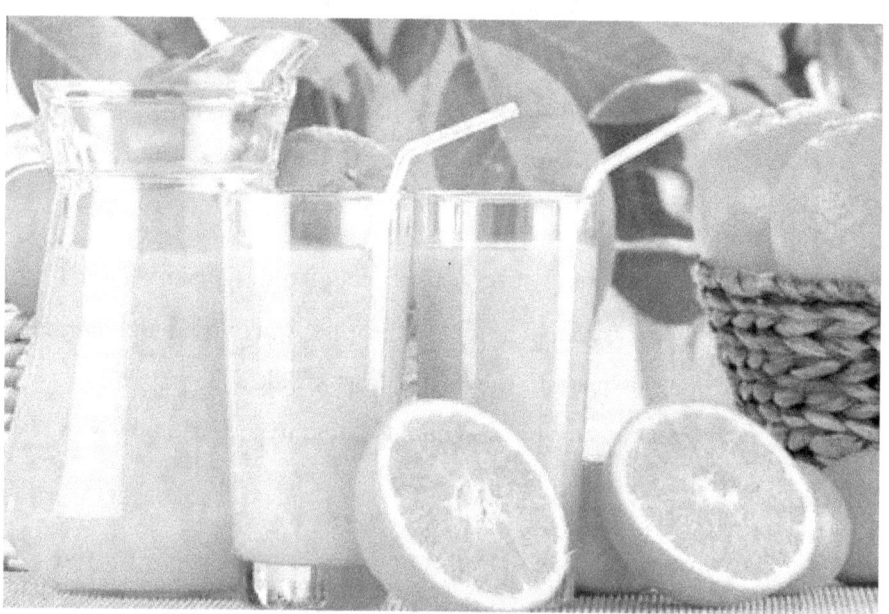

Water Therapy

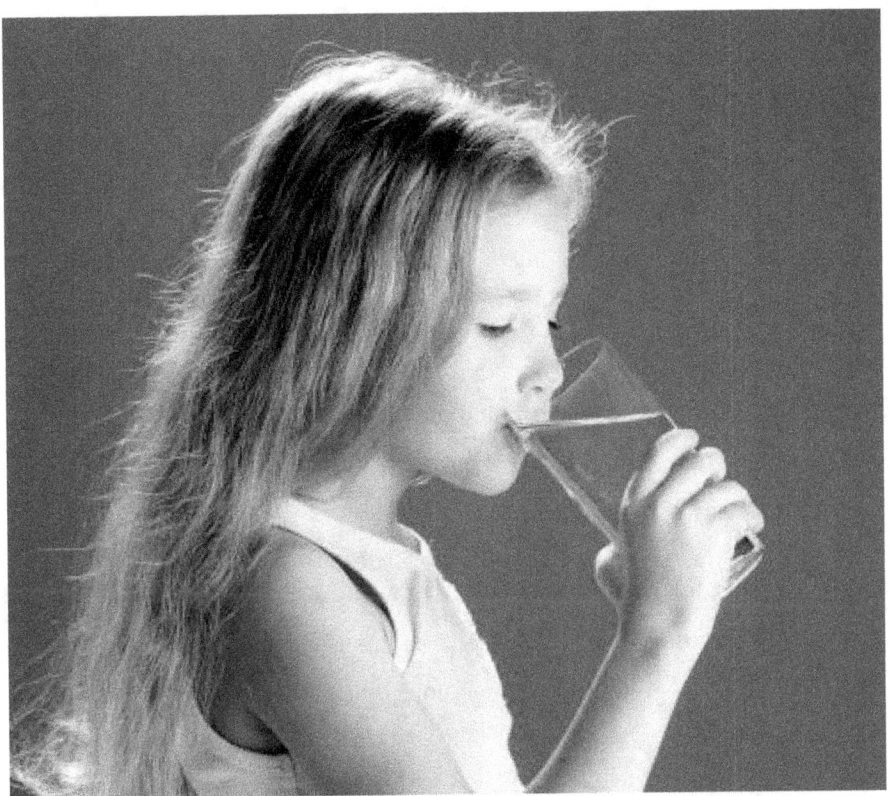

Try this water therapy out if you are suffering from chronic constipation. Take a glassful of hot water at a temperature which you are able to tolerate and drink it in small sips.[1] This should be drunk after you have eaten your

---

[1] Reminds me of the fact that people are able to drink boiling hot coffee and boiling hot tea or soup, but they cannot drink boiling hot water! Astonishing what the mind allows you to accept and not to accept!

meal. You can also take some warm/hot water and drink it in sips, along with your meal. Drink a glass of water, first thing in the morning when you wake up.[2]

Also I found someone doing something rather amusing for people suffering from a sluggish digestive system. This is called the wet bandage treatment. First, you need to massage the stomach area with some warm olive oil, coconut oil or mustard oil. Any Sherlock Holmes is going to tell you that this is to get the muscles moving, especially if you live a sedentary lifestyle. After that, take some wet cloths or bandages, and place them on the stomach. Leave them on to reactivate your system. I also saw some people being treated to a traditional wet mud on the stomach treatment. This was then covered with a cloth and left overnight. This is considered to be a sure fire cure for constipation.

If you are interested in this treatment, you would want to know the mud used in such treatments. They are called mudpacks and are of different types. This URL is going to give you more information on this subject.

http://naturopathycure.com/Mud-Therapy-Benefits.php

Anyway, the mud, I saw being plastered on to the stomach of a person suffering from constipation had been gathered from the bottom of the nearest river! And it worked perfectly. In fact, in Africa, even to this day, mud packs and mud baths are done with the help of mud gathered from the nearest water source.

---

[2] I have been doing that for the last 15 years – half a bottle of water kept on my bedside table – and I do not suffer from constipation because my system gets cleared within half an hour.

This mud is also used for wrapping up pieces of food and meat which is then baked slowly in a wood fire.[3]

Irregular Bowel Movement Habits

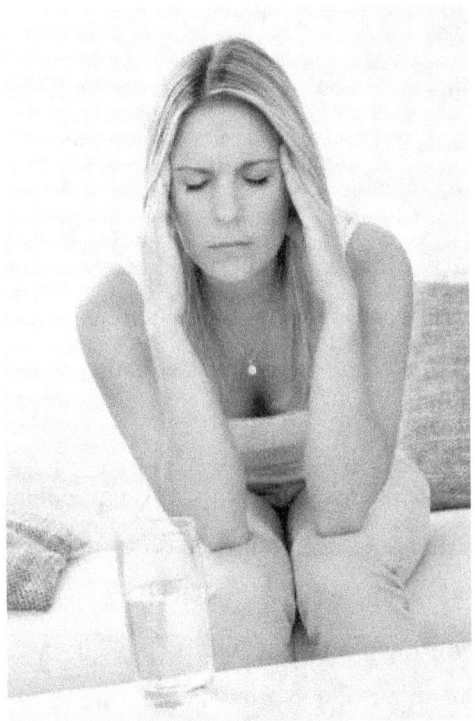

---

[3] It is of course a delicious meal, based on personal experience. You remove the mud and eat the perfectly cooked morsel inside. This process is also followed in many parts of the East where you can consider this to be clay cooking. This reminds me of the story of one of those young bluebloods who were told to go shoot in Africa for the peace of their family and society in London. He was invited to one of the tribal get-togethers where he was offered this mud baked feast. He refused it. Lord Lah di dah did not eat the food cooked in his club because it was not up to his expectations. They did not expect him to eat savage food baked in a mud oven, covered with mud.

One does not know his future fate. But he never came back from Africa. One could devoutly wish that he was consumed, well wrapped up in mud and baked in a clay pot, just because of his narrowminded and insular snobbishness and rudeness. But alas, cannibalism in many parts of the world, including Africa had been stamped out in the nineteenth century.

You will be surprised to know that there are number of people who have the tendency of not going to the bathroom, the moment they feel some pressure on their bowels. When asked why they are not eliminating the waste, even though they are feeling the discomfort of that pressure, they say that waiting for an hour or more will mean more waste collected and more waste eliminated in one go itself.

This is a specious and erroneous idea. They cannot understand that during that one hour, the body is getting subjected to even more toxins which should have been removed as soon as possible.

In many parts of the world today, and even in ancient times, a baby was and is potty trained with a verbal autosuggestion command of *siii-siiii- siiiii* by the mother, about an hour after every meal, and also early in the morning when he wakes up.

I do not know the mental reasoning behind this particular sound effect, but this is the practice which has been followed down the ages and this can be considered to be a very simple and effective way of teaching a child to go in for regular bowel movement without "postponing" its natural eliminating process. In fact, when the children grow up to be adults, they get into the habit of emptying their bowels in the morning. And so they feel "lighter", more energetic and healthier.

On the other hand, there are people who are so busy doing other duties, that they decide to postpone the urge to empty out their bowels. I remember a really amusing incident when I was training at management school. We had come to visit a factory as a part of our practical training in order to see how it worked, the process, the human resource development, the administration, the finances, and so on.

One of my friends did not seem so enthusiastic and kept wriggling. It seemed she was in too much of a hurry that morning to go to the bathroom, because she thought that she did not need to. And now at midday, her stomach had started protesting. Being a lady, she was too shy to ask the males around her whether there was a bathroom in the vicinity. And she had this lowering feeling that possibly that bathroom would be a male bathroom, because there were no female workers visible in that particular area of the factory!

I still remember her discomfort, the faces she made and how miserable she looked. Luckily, our professor was a sensible sort of person, and asked her what the matter was. She was too shy to confess that she needed to go to the bathroom and fast. Luckily, another friend who was not so particular about modesty and shyness piped up immediately – "upset stomach, sir, too much pizza and hamburgers last night."

Somehow this explanation was more acceptable than saying that one needed to go to the bathroom because one had not "been" that morning! So life is like that!

P. was immediately shown into the CEO's Italian marble tiled bathroom, the glory of which she described to us in hushed whispers when she came out "relieved". Somehow all of us decided that we had upset stomachs and we had to go inspect that luxuriously appointed bathroom and I would not be surprised if the CEO was not pleased at our scarcely hidden appreciative faces when we came out of that luxurious room.

But remember that you may not be so lucky as we were and that is why if you are suffering from constipation and you are going out on a trip somewhere, do not take any product before hand, which promises to clear up your system for you. It means that you might find yourself in an embarrassing situation, with absolutely no recourse or access to a bathroom. This gets doubly embarrassing, if you are female, because you cannot retreat behind the nearest wall or bush insouciantly or with impunity.

Sedentary Lifestyles

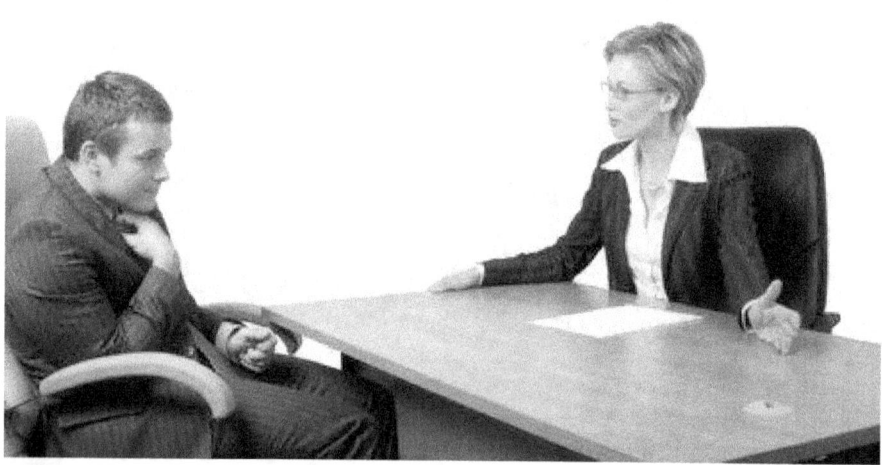

I noticed that since I took up a desk job, and I had to sit piloting a desk and using my brains more than doing any sort of physical effort, I started to suffer from constipation. Now, why was this so? Here is some sort of explanation, which I decided for myself.

On my desk job, harried with schedules and meetings, I did not bother much about eating meals regularly. I often dined off a sandwich on my office desk when throughout my life I had been eating properly cooked meals at breakfast time, lunchtime, and dinnertime, on my dinner table at regular hours.

Besides this, the only exercise I did was going from one conference table to another meeting, from one floor to the other via lift. I did not bother climbing up the stairs because 14 stories were definitely not my cup of tea. Only Hollywood heroes pursuing villains ran up and down staircases without breaking into a sweat or collapsing, calling for an ambulance. I was definitely not that heroic sort.

So I sat in front of my computer and my overloaded desk in a crumpled up position not moving for hours. My posture was abominable. My upper torso was nearly touching my lower torso, because my shoulders were rounded and I was all hunched up in my chair.

Naturally, apart from the pressure on my lungs, which did not get enough of oxygen, my stomach also began to feel this pressure. The muscles in that particular region did not get any chance to expand, which would have been their normal norm, if I was doing some physical work outdoors.

This sedentary lifestyle without any sort of exercise immediately began to show results in the form of gaining weight, bad posture, spondylitis, and, of course, constipation. And then I remembered something my father had said which his father had told him. Nobody in their area suffered from constipation, because they kept working from dawn to dusk. The stomach got plenty of exercise and when it was digesting food, the motion of the body doing some sort of exercise kept all its muscles working properly and in a healthy manner.

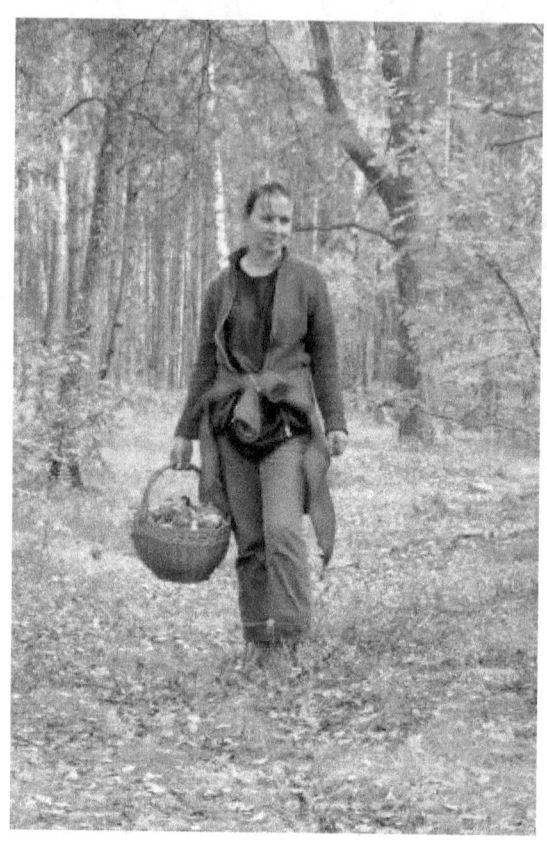

Anything done outdoors, including walking is going to help your heart, body, mind, soul, and spirit grow healthier and heal itself.

Any rare person suffering from constipation in that particular area was immediately put to work on the fields. He was then given plenty of water/buttermilk to drink whenever he felt thirsty. Apart from this, he was given water at dawn, so that he would have a healthy bowel movement, by the time he was ready to wake up fully in about 2 hours time. The moment he woke up, he was given more water to drink. By this time, his bowels would be ready to eliminate the waste accumulated during the night. Also, he was given water to drink one hour before eating his lunch in the afternoon and one hour before he went to sleep.

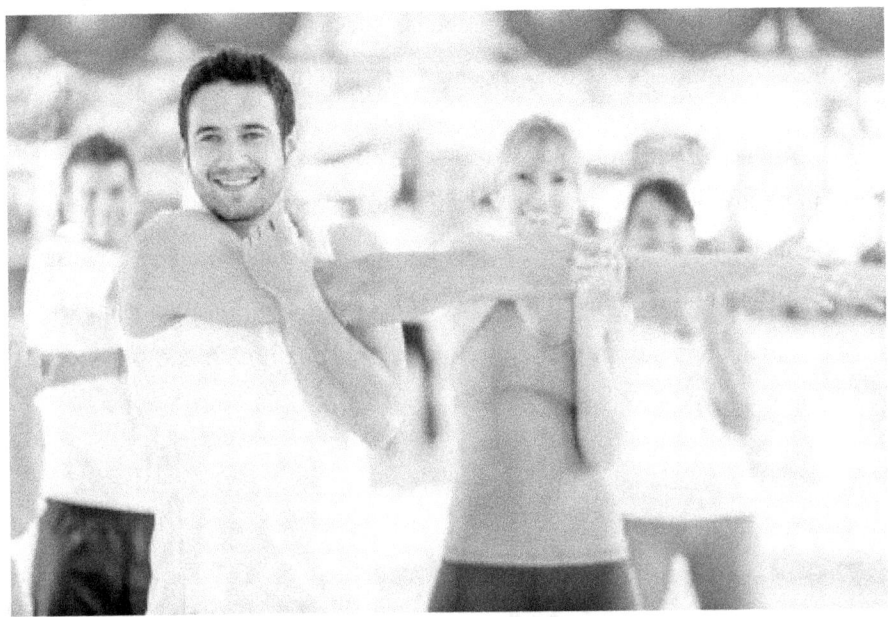

Physical workouts several days a week, are also good to keep your system toned and healthy.

Try this out, because this is an ancient remedy to keep your system working properly. Naturally, my father never suffered from constipation. Also, he put me into the habit of placing 2 L (half a gallon) of water by my bedside. I wake up at least 2 times in the night and have a deep drink of water. By the time I wake up in the morning, my systems are ready to go, and I clear them out before a shower. So naturally, this is what I tell my friends, suffering from constipation – drink plenty of water morning, noon, and night.

Factors Encouraging Constipation

Do you know that many of us encourage constipation through sheer ignorance? That is because we are weakening our system with the intake of tobacco, tea, alcohol, and other stimulants. These stimulants are quite capable of changing our natural biochemistry and that is why you may find yourself suffering more from constipation.

Also, there are plenty of medicines, which are given for high blood pressure and for heart diseases. Some of them are calcium channel blockers. These include Nifedipine which you may buy as Procardia.Amlodipine is another such drug which is normally used to treat angina and high blood pressure. It is sold in the market as Norvasc.

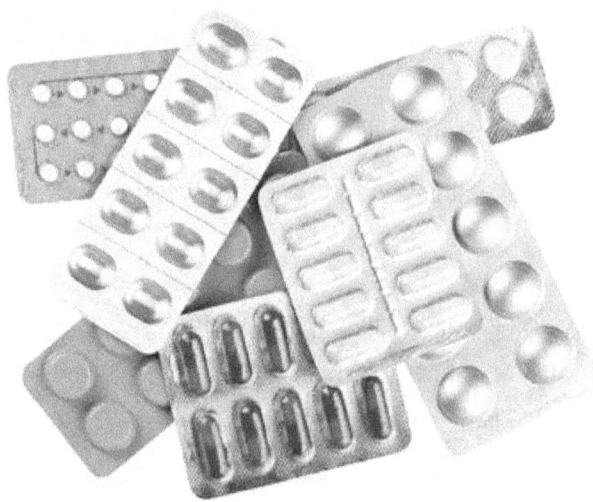

Are these prescribed drugs causing constipation in you?

These are some medicines which can cause constipation as a side effect. Also, you may not know that the tonics which you take to treat coughs and colds like codeine have Poppy based extracts in them. These are going to promote constipation. Also, if you are suffering from anemia, you are going to be given iron tablets. This mineral may improve your RBC count, but it is going to have a constipatory effect on your digestive system.

You may want to ask your doctor about the side effects of the drugs prescribed to you, especially if you are suffering from chronic constipation.

Apart from these factors, there are other factors which can cause or promote constipation. Most of us are too impatient to let nature take its own course and allow the elimination of waste products at its own given time. We want to hasten up the process by taking laxatives and products which interfere with the natural working of the digestive system.

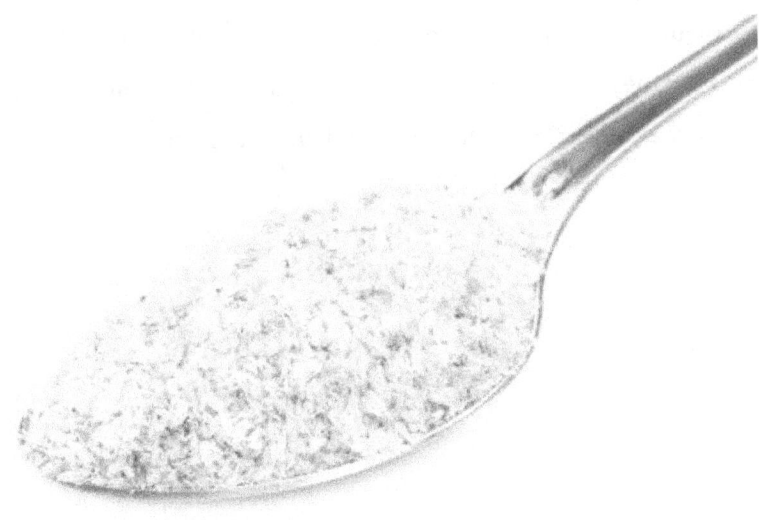

Powdered psyllium.

I know about a person who is so worried about constipation that she takes Isabgol husk every morning with breakfast so that she can be assured of "relief" sometime during the day.

This is an artificial way of forcing your system to empty itself out. If you persist on doing this, your digestive system and intestines are going to stop functioning in their normal manner. They are going to lose an up and grow weak. A regular consumption of such medicines can also cause piles.

So now you are going to get ancient time-tested methods on how you can prevent constipation and cure it. Remember that all of them are natural, and they can be taken without any worry about side effects. So choose the remedy which best suits you, and get rid of that constipation worry once and for all.

Constipation is not an ailment in itself. It is brought about by a disturbance or an irregularity in your daily routine. That is why, if you want to get rid of constipation, never take a laxative. It is going to weaken your natural system, and also interfere with the natural eliminating processes of your body.

Curing Constipation Naturally

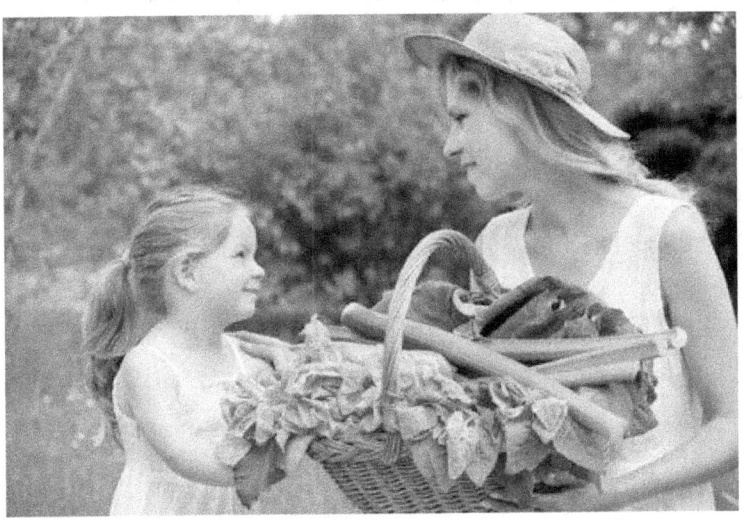

Start eating more of raw fruit and vegetables. The ancients lived on a diet of fruit, vegetable, nuts, and roots with meat eaten only occasionally. And they lived long and fruitful lives. As time went by, lifestyles and eating habits started to change, with more of proteinaceous matter and lesser of vegetable and fruit matter being eaten.

This proteinaceous food, especially if it was in the shape of red meat was harder to digest. And by the time it was digested a second meal was already ingested. So the stomach was hard put to digest to such heavy meals without any fruits and vegetables to supply the fiber which would help in the elimination process.

And so people started suffering more from constipation. And they began to look at remedies to prevent that instead of taking more care about their diet.

They tried to prevent constipation by eating onions, along with the meat, and so you need to add at least one raw onion to every meal.

In medieval and Regency England onions were considered to be food eaten only by the lower classes and garlic as something eaten by their natural enemies, the Frenchmen![4] That is why the aristocracy was more susceptible to illnesses because they were not going to eat a lower-class diet, which included onions and cabbages. They had no resistance, and any disease carried them off like flies dying in the heat.

But they did not understand that all that could be prevented with the eating of more green vegetables including onions. Also, they suffered greatly from constipation, because their diet was rich in meat, lots of alcohol and rich spicy food. This caused acidity and also dyspepsia. They also suffered a lot from the gout because of their unhealthy diet.

---

[4] Their pejorative terms for the French was *garlic eater* and *frog eater*, at that time. The French retaliated by calling them *rosbif* or roast beef.

Diet

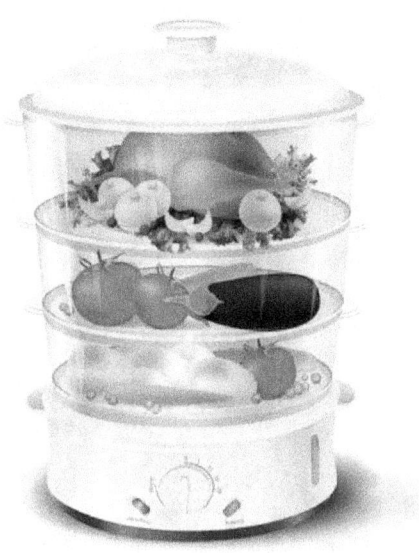

Steam cooked and boiled food is easier to digest, when compared to fried food.

Try this diet out now. It has been in use for millenniums, and is the best way in which you can prevent and heal constipation. Eat sprouts, and pulses with their skins, sprouted grain is also good. Boil your vegetables before you eat them. You can also steam them.

Green vegetables eaten best steamed, cooked, or raw are going to keep your system very healthy. Salads should be an integral part of every meal. These should include green vegetables and red vegetables including lettuce, cucumber, tomatoes and even green onions.

Ripe Guavas

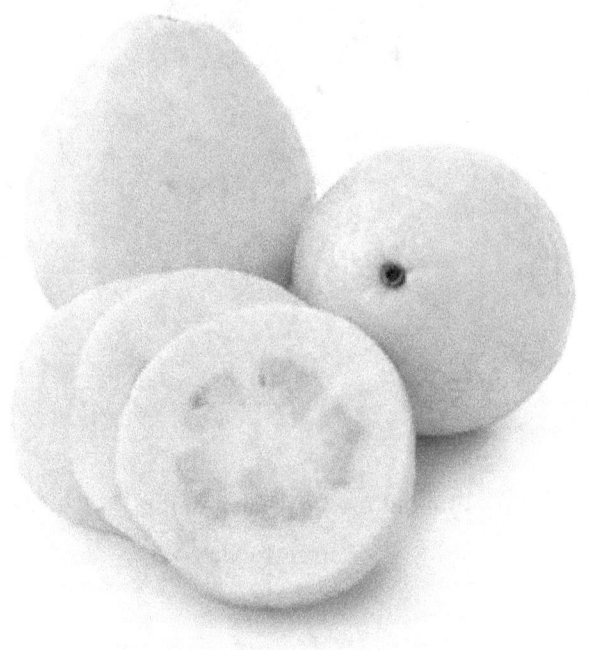

Try spinach juice, oranges, lemons, mango, papayas, and guavas in your meal, if available. When I was a child, we lived in an area, where papayas, gooseberries and guavas grew so profusely, that we kids did not want to touch them, even though our father used to make tempting *Mmmm, this is*

delicious, this tastes so good noises, whenever he cut into a ripe orange papaya at every meal time.

According to us, what he found sweet and delicious was boring, because we had so many papayas along with other fruit growing in the garden. When he found that we had begun treating the guavas also to this casual neglecting attitude, he tried another psychological stunt.

He described the round seeds in guavas as little rollers in our stomachs. They would go rolling all around our stomachs, and cause the contents to move. They were pushy, bossy, and quite mean little rollers. And they pushed everything out of our stomachs, the next morning.[5]

We found that particular description fascinating and that is why we began to eat as many guavas as we could, off the trees, visualizing the bossy little rollers doing their activity in our stomachs

. What we did not notice is that father never ate them; he did not find them delicious and he did not like the seeds sticking in or between his teeth![6]

Anybody suffering from constipation should remember that guavas should be eaten before you eat your meal. If you eat guavas after lunch or dinner,

---

[5] We kids were about 7 and 4 at that time and that is why we enjoyed this descriptive story very much! Even today, whenever I eat okra and guavas, I have to smile at the rollers, which incidentally are still doing their work of preventing constipation!

[6] You could say that he could enjoy the guavas by removing all the seeds beforehand. But plain ripe guava pulp is rather bland, boring, and dull without lots of salt, pepper and spices sprinkled on it to make it a bit more interesting.

they are going to cause constipation! Try eating them for breakfast. And if you are suffering from chronic constipation, eat them twice a day.

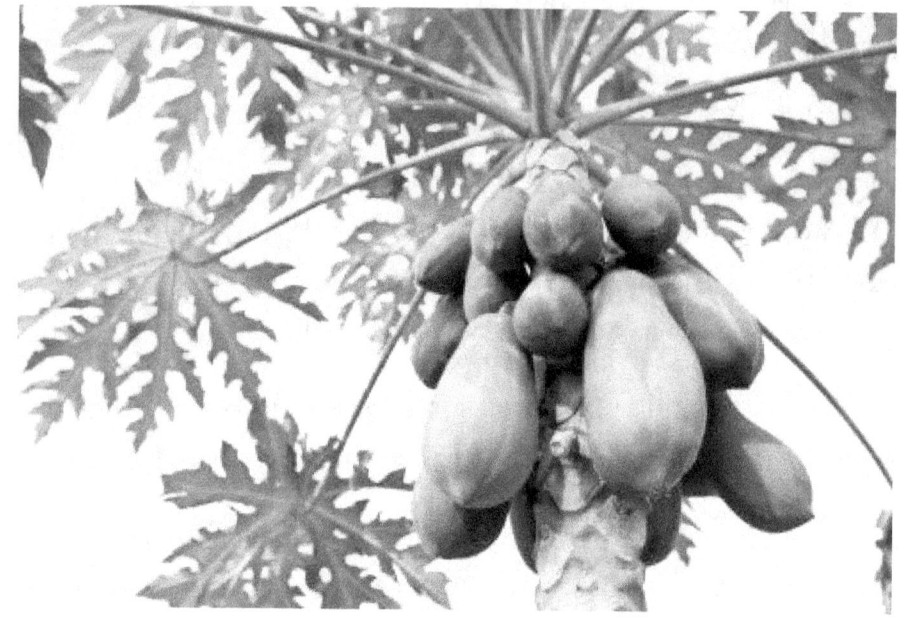

Papaya tree.

As for papayas, they should be eaten at night before you go to sleep the next morning you are going to have your system clear and regular.

Along with that, try increasing the fiber content in your food. Try eating porridge, coarsely ground flour with the bran in, and stop eating refined flour items like cake, bread, and pasta. However, if the pasta is made up of ground and unrefined wheat flour, then papaya tree papaya you can enjoy it.

Fruits have plenty of fiber but you cannot get that fiber in the fruit juice. So drink the fruit juice only to keep yourself well dehydrated and eat the fruit pulp for its fiber content.

Why are laxatives harmful? As I told you before, laxatives interfere with the normal natural processes of your body. I remember an elder complaining to me that he took laxatives and that would help him have a regular bowel movement. But after some time that laxative had begun to stop having such an excellent effect. He could not have a regular bowel movement, even when he applied "pressure." Well, the laxatives had done their work of spoiling the regular system and themselves had stopped working. So this is what is going to happen in the long run. Your system is going to get so accustomed to laxatives that it is not going to work on its own. And when the laxatives stop working, you are literally up ordure creek without a paddle.

So that is why do not get into the habit of taking any sort of laxatives ever.

Carrots and Citrus Fruits

Carrots and citrus fruits are excellent preventative and curative measures for constipation. Take 250 g (half pound) of carrots, chop them up, and eat them first thing in the morning before you have your breakfast. You will need to chew them well. Not only are they going to clear your system, but they are going to make you feel hungrier throughout the day.

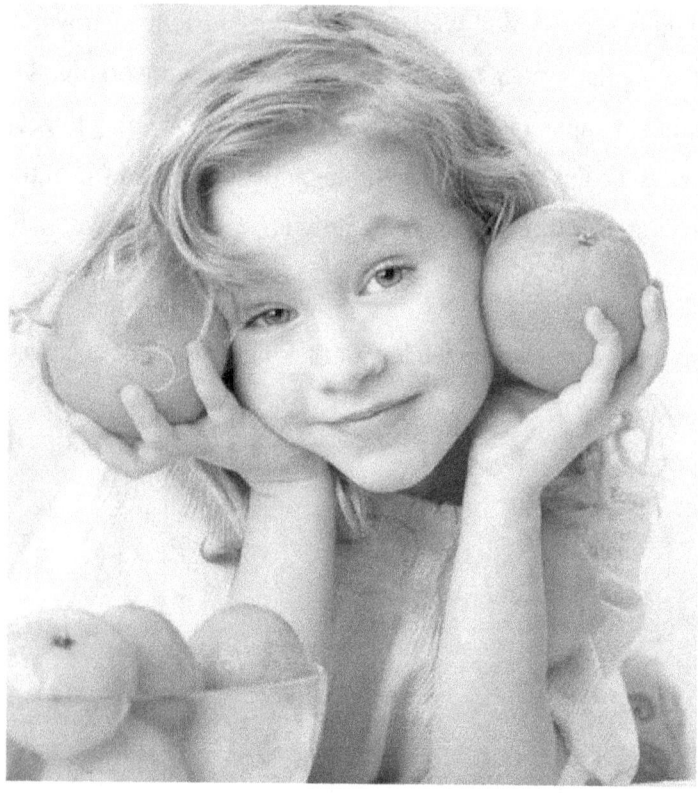

Anybody suffering from chronic constipation can be cured with the help of lemons. Just take lemon juice with warm water before you go to sleep. This is going to clear up your stomach in the morning. 1 and a half teaspoons full of lemon juice and one spoonful of honey can also be added to one glass of water and drank before you go to sleep. This gets rid of chronic constipation.

Have an orange for breakfast. Apart from giving you your daily dose of vitamin C, it is going to help cure constipation. Along with that, take a glass of fresh orange juice. Try this for a week. This is also going to improve your digestive system and strengthen it.

Gooseberries

Gooseberries are about the best source of vitamin C that I know. As a child, it was a part of our school life that we friends had to get gooseberries and raw guavas from the trees growing in our gardens and share them with the rest of our friends in order to show our loyalty, solidarity and friendship. This daily diet of gooseberries when we were kids had an excellent long-term effect on our general health.

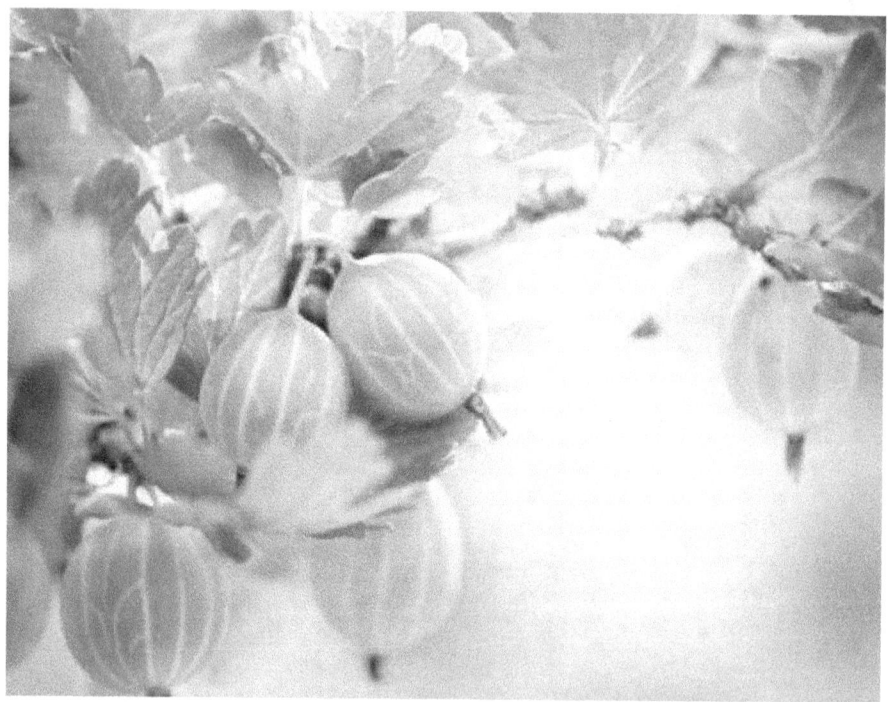

We had a very strong immunity system, and a very strong digestive system. It has lasted for more than 4 decades and has kept us healthy and able to survive in disease ridden areas as well as eat all sort of fares without succumbing to botulism or upset stomachs.

Along with that, all of us had shining and glowing skins without any pimples and blemishes, when we hit our teens. Also, our hair was long, glossy and lustrous. Incidentally, gooseberries are considered to be one of the most important beauty products in the East for hair care.

Eating raw gooseberries is an acquired taste, because they are horribly sour. But we enjoyed them with salt and liked the sweet taste of salt and sour, the moment it touched our tongues! That in itself was something really wondrous to us children.

So if you are suffering from any sort of chronic constipation, try eating some raw gooseberries throughout the day. At night, take one teaspoonful of gooseberry powder with either water or with warm milk. This is a natural cure for chronic constipation.

Apples

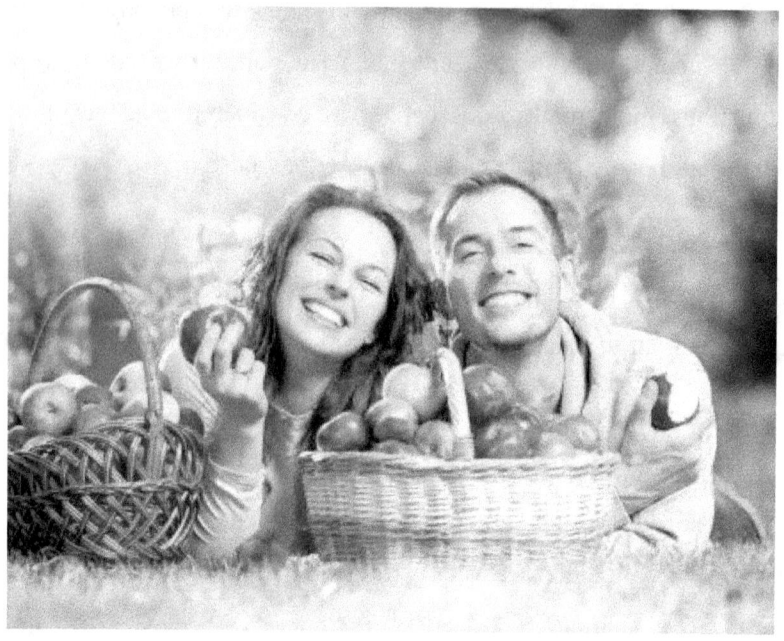

An apple a day keeps the doctor away. It also keeps constipation away. But remember that you always have to eat the apple on an empty stomach. If you eat it after meals, you are going to suffer from constipation! Remember the guavas? If you are suffering from chronic constipation, do not peel the apple before you eat it. However, if you are suffering from dysentery or diarrhea, remove the peel before you eat the apple.

Conclusion

This book has given you plenty of information about constipation, its prevention, its symptoms, and its natural cure.

A number of people are going to tell me that they swear by psyllium husks, which is also known as isabgol. This is a fiber derived from a Plantago ovata plant. Any sort of laxative is not something that I am going to advise, but people persist on taking this fiber because they said that their system works only when they take this for breakfast.

Well, if you take 2 teaspoons full of psyllium husks powder in warm water or warm milk, at breakfast time, it is going to help you a lot. But you may soon find yourself taking up to 4 teaspoons full of this husk, to get your system moving. Well! Also, you may find yourself suffering from bloating. Now, why does this happen? That is because this husk is going to cause gas and flatulence in the stomach. This is due to the activity of stomach bacteria on the psyllium husk.

In such cases, you will need to reduce your dose of psyllium or stop taking it altogether.

This husk is capable of soaking up all the water in your intestines. This is going to increase the quantity of solid fecal matter there. This means that your system begins to move towards elimination from the bowels. This is what makes people think that this husk is extremely helpful in cases of constipation.

So here are some tips when you are taking psyllium husk. Drink water, 2 or 3 times after you have taken the dose at breakfast. This is going to cause the husk to swell up properly. This is also why, this is never taken at night, before you go to sleep but always in the daytime, especially after breakfast. Take it immediately after your meal.

Now that I have given you the best natural cure and solutions for constipation, you will never have to suffer it again!

Live Long and Prosper!

Author Bio

Dueep Jyot Singh is a Management and IT Professional who managed to gather Postgraduate qualifications in Management and English and Degrees in Science, French and Education while pursuing different enjoyable career options like being an hospital administrator, IT,SEO and HRD Database Manager/ trainer, movie , radio and TV scriptwriter, theatre artiste and public speaker, lecturer in French, Marketing and Advertising, ex-Editor of Hearts On Fire (now known as Solstice) Books Missouri USA, advice columnist and cartoonist, publisher and Aviation School trainer, ex-moderator on Medico.in, banker, student councilor ,travelogue writer … among other things!

One fine morning, she decided that she had enough of killing herself by Degrees and went back to her first love -- writing. It's more enjoyable! She already has 48 published academic and 14 fiction- in- different- genre books under her belt.

When she is not designing websites or making Graphic design illustrations for clients , she is browsing through old bookshops hunting for treasures, of which she has an enviable collection – including R.L. Stevenson, O.Henry, Dornford Yates, Maurice Walsh, De Maupassant, Victor Hugo, Sapper, C.N. Williamson, "Bartimeus" and the crown of her collection- Dickens "The Old Curiosity Shop," and "Martin Chuzzlewit" and so on… Just call her "Renaissance Woman") - collecting herbal remedies, acting like Universal Helping Hand/Agony Aunt, or escaping to her dear mountains for a bit of exploring, collecting herbs and plants and trekking.

Check out some of the other JD-Biz Publishing books

Gardening Series on Amazon

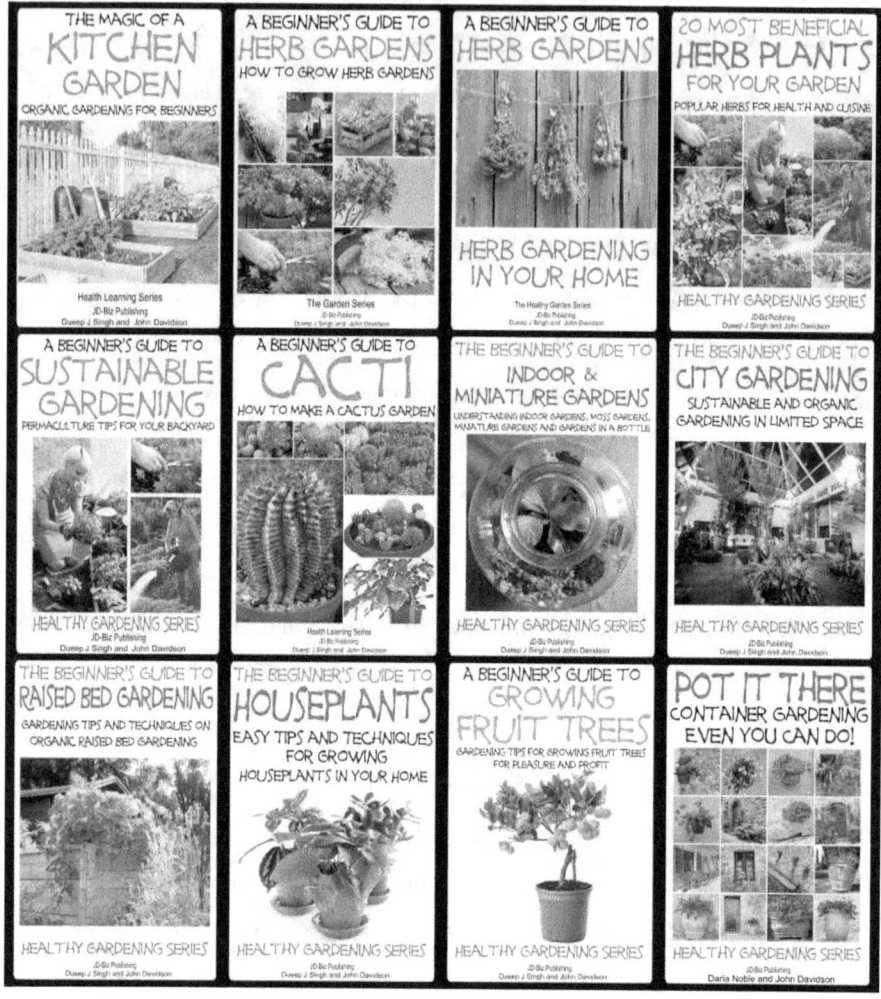

Health Learning Series

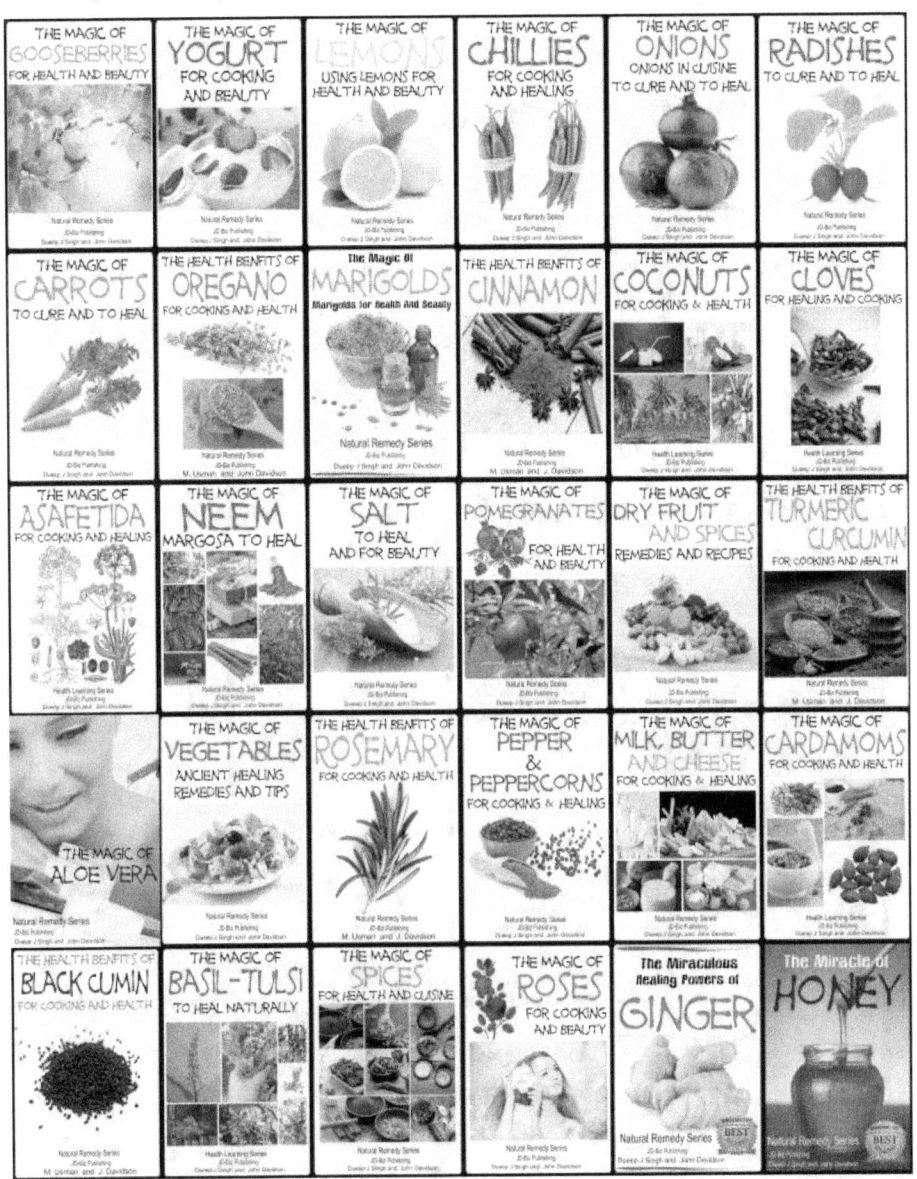

Country Life Books

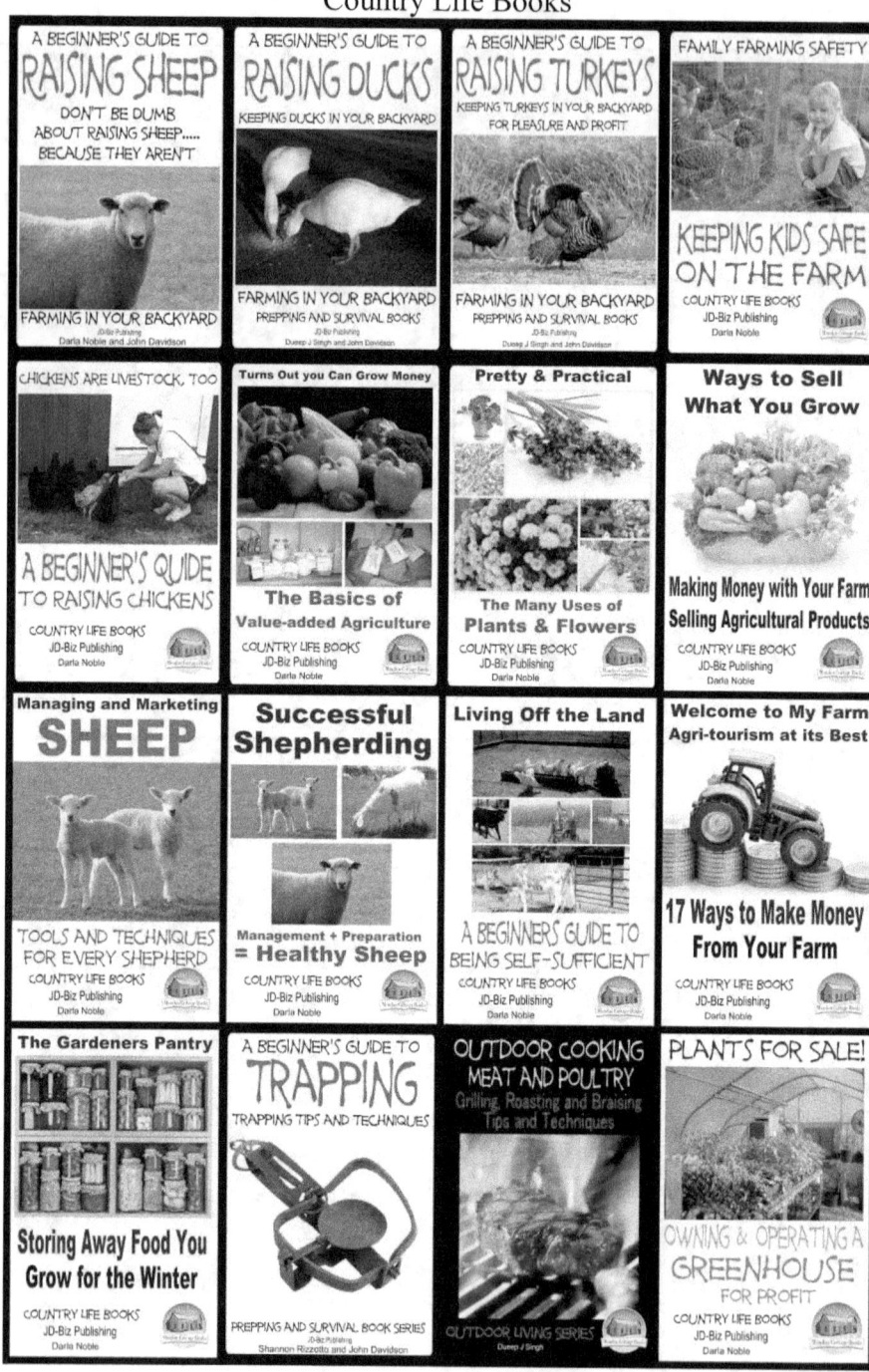

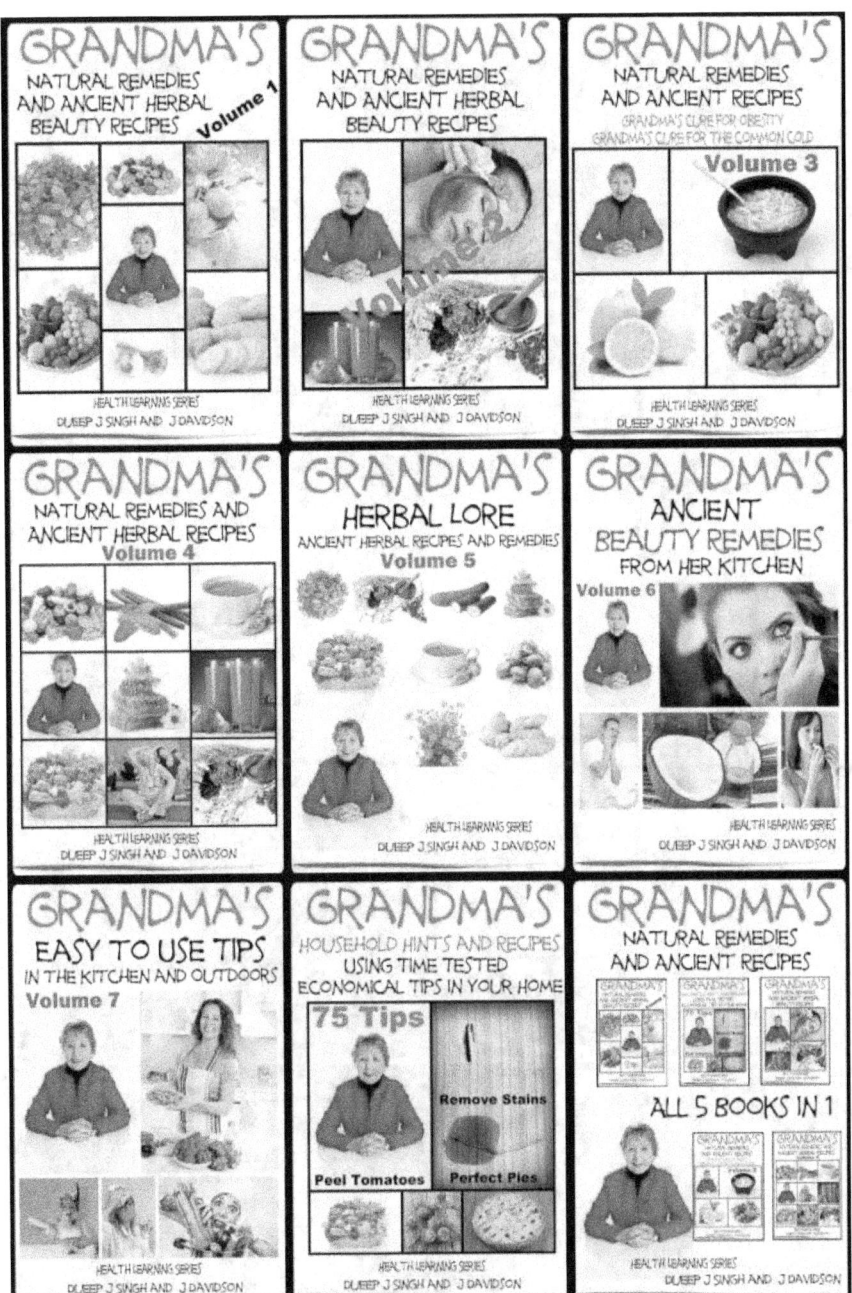

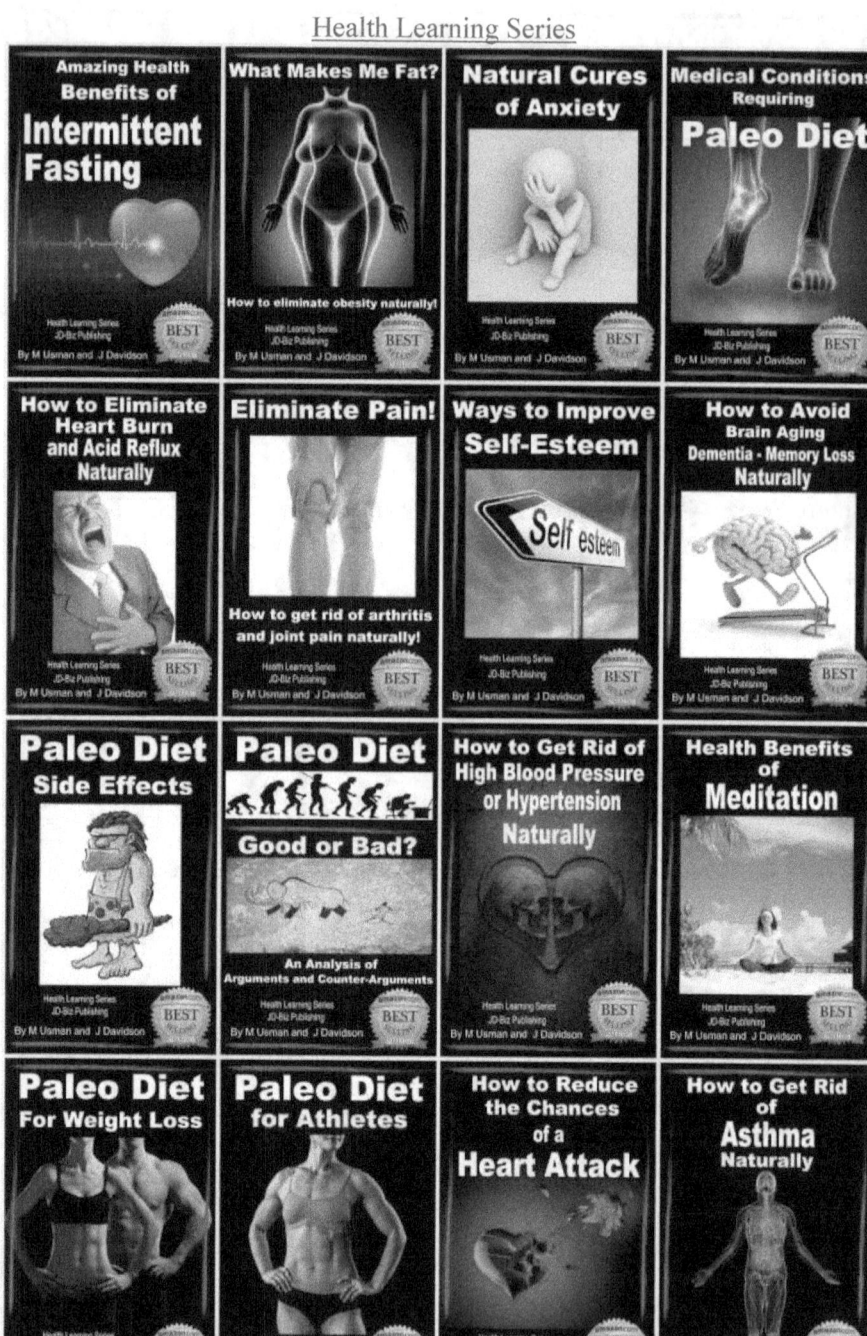

Natural Cures for Constipation

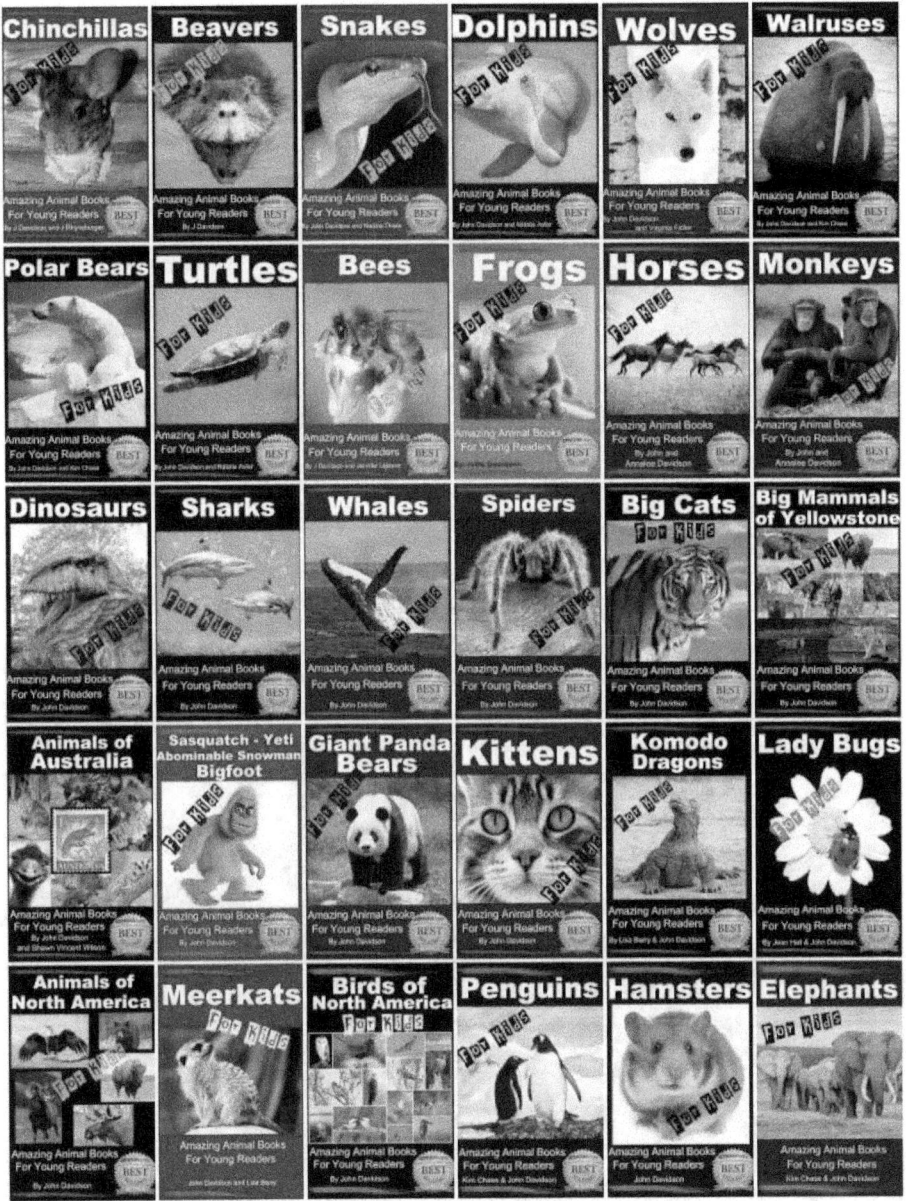

Learn To Draw Series

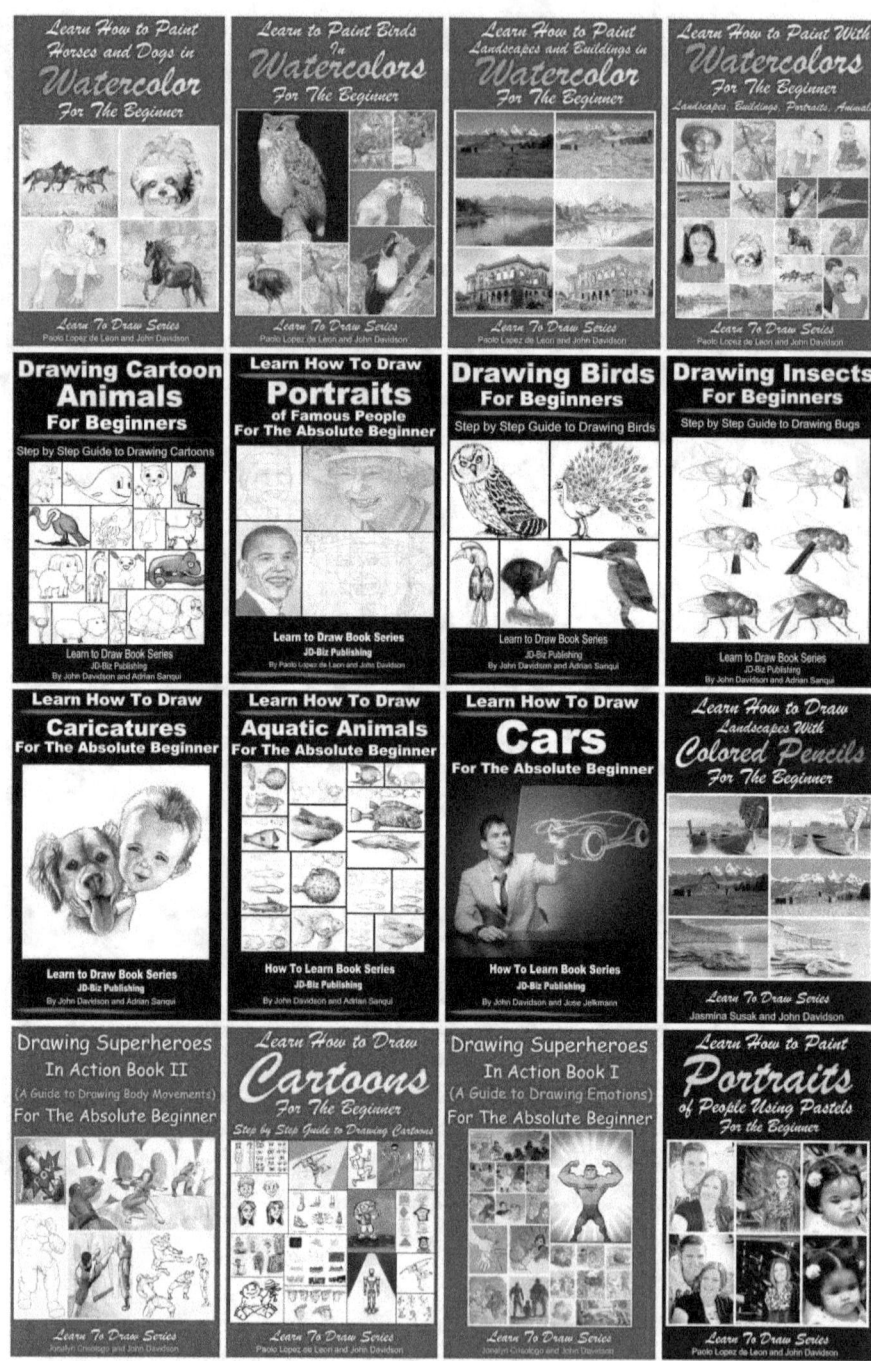

How to Build and Plan Books

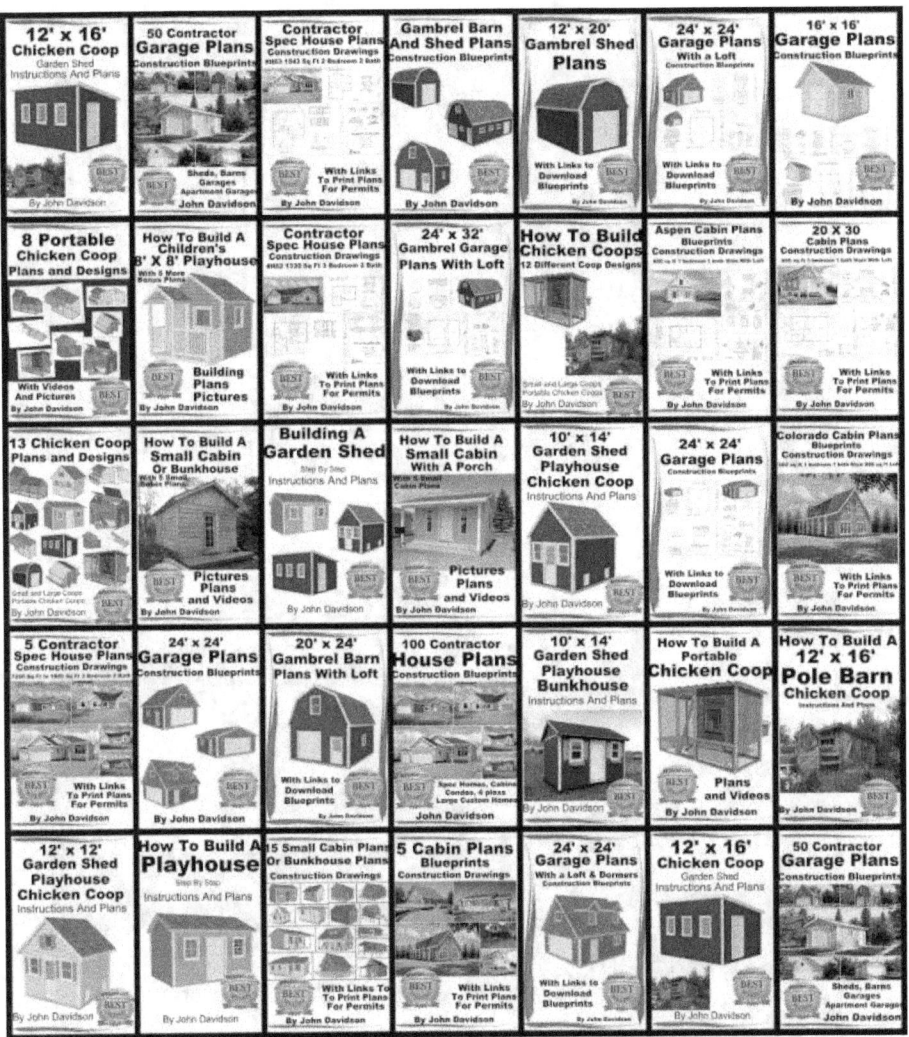

Entrepreneur Book Series

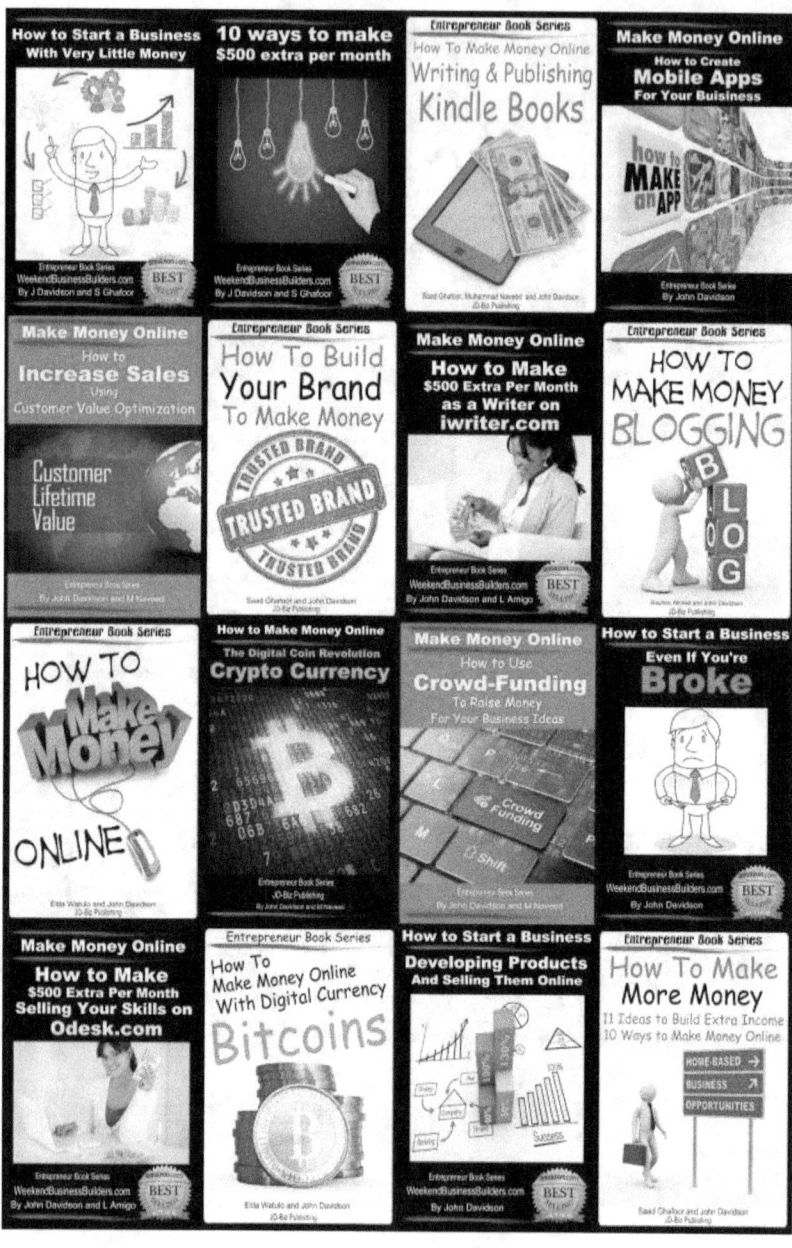

Our books are available at

1. Amazon.com

2. Barnes and Noble

3. Itunes

4. Kobo

5. Smashwords

6. Google Play Books

Publisher

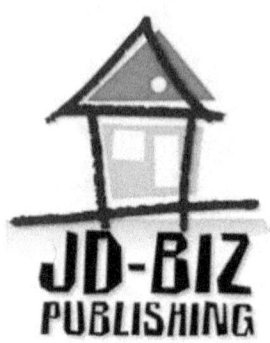

JD-Biz Corp

P O Box 374

Mendon, Utah 84325

http://www.jd-biz.com/

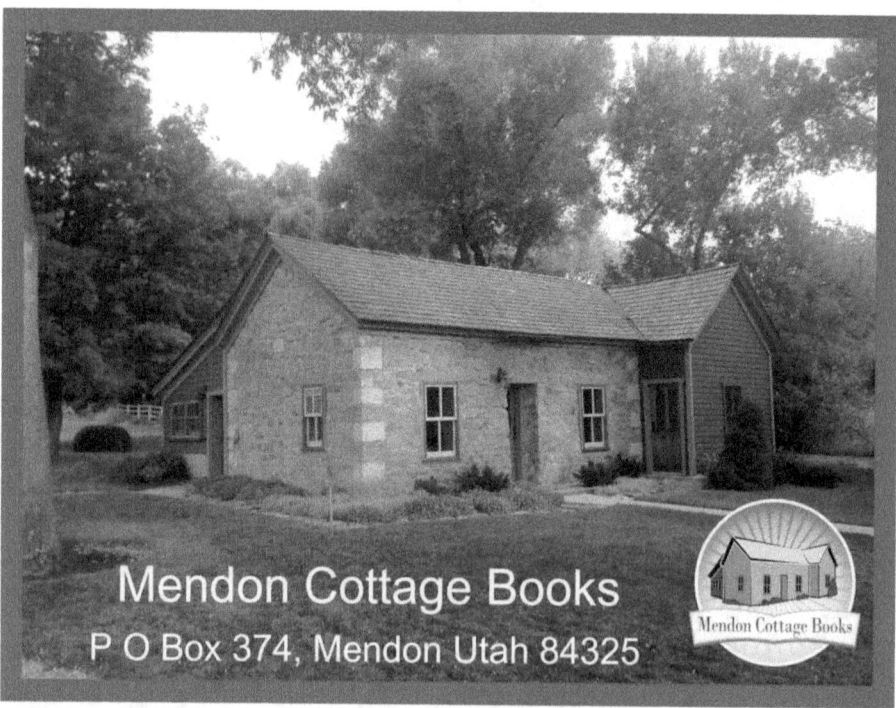

Mendon Cottage Books

P O Box 374, Mendon Utah 84325